The Harcombe Diet®

For Men

Published by Columbus Publishing Ltd 2011
www.columbuspublishing.co.uk

ISBN 978-1-907797-12-5

A CIP record of this book is available from the British Library.

Cover design by Lewis Kokoc

The content of this book is intended to inform, entertain and provoke your
thinking. This is not intended as medical advice. It may, however, make you
question current medical and nutritional advice. That's your choice. It's your
life and health in your hands. Neither the author nor the publisher can be held
responsible or liable for any loss or claim arising from the use, or misuse, of
the content of this book.

COLUMBUS PUBLISHING

Contents

		Page
Introduction		**2**
Part One: For Starters		**5**
1	What is The Harcombe Diet®?	**6**
2	How is it different to other diets?	**8**
3	What can you eat?	**10**
Part Two: The Main Course		**11**
4	Phase 1 – The five day 'kick-start' plan, for rapid weight loss	**12**
5	Phase 2 – The weight-loss plan, for eating real food, in unlimited quantities, while losing weight and gaining health	**21**
6	Phase 3 – The way-of-life plan, for eating what you want, while staying at your fighting weight	**45**
Part Three: Dessert (optional)		**49**
7	The three conditions that cause overweight	**50**
8	"The Viagra Principle"	**52**
9	Fitness and nutrition	**54**
10	Eating out and losing weight	**56**
11	Cholesterol, fat and health (*)	**59**
12	Did you know?	**64**
Glossary, Shopping List & Index		**66**

(*) If you read just one of the optional chapters, this is the one recommended.

The Glossary has simple definitions of all the terms used in the book. If you don't know your fats from your carbs, or what insulin has got to do with your waistline, check them out.

The Harcombe Diet®

For Men

"We want to be slim.

Our motivation is not in question.

The advice we are being given most certainly is."

To find out more...

www.zoeharcombe.com

www.theharcombedietformen.com

www.theharcombedietclub.com

www.theobesityepidemic.org

Introduction

Men...

The human body is the true wonder of the world. We have 206 bones and all the muscles and ligaments needed to move this complex structure with suppleness, stamina and strength. Some men can run 100 metres in fewer than 10 seconds. Others can run a marathon in just over two hours. The heart is one of the most reliable pumps on earth. It will beat approximately 70 times a minute, 60 minutes an hour, 24 hours a day, 365 days a year for 76 years.

The average man is 5'9" and weighs 172lbs. On average, 43% of this is muscle, 14% fat, 14% bone and marrow, 12% internal organs, 9% connective tissue and skin and 8% blood. Water is in all of these body parts, from muscle to blood, so, overall, Mr Average is approximately 50-60% water. The largest organ in the body (steady on) is the skin – laid out flat it would cover a king size bed sheet. There are approximately 100,000 hairs on a man. Finally, and most importantly for the human race, man can produce 3,000 sperm a second and lose 200-300 million with each ejaculation.

Our bodies repair themselves and fight life-threatening infection. They digest food efficiently and manage their own waste production. We can fly to the moon, cause, or prevent, the extinction of other species, laugh, cry and play poker. We are truly remarkable. Perhaps the most remarkable feature of the human being, however, is its survival mechanism – the body will do whatever it takes to keep us alive.

Man and our ancestors have been trying to store food and survive for 3,500,000 years and, only in the last few decades, has man been trying to lose weight. So, here's a question – do you want this incredibly powerful machine, the human body, working *with* you or *against* you, when you're trying to lose weight?

... and cars

If a car mechanic told you to drive from California to New York, with only enough petrol to get to Iowa, let alone to flog the car even harder, so that it would only get to Colorado, you would think he was mad and yet millions of people in the 'developed' world are deliberately trying to run their bodies on less fuel than they need, every single day.

The vast majority of diets are based on this advice – they're trying to get you to eat less (diet) and/or do more (exercise). You wouldn't do this to you car – why would you do it to your body?

... and not enough fuel

If you try to eat less the body doesn't know you've started a diet, it thinks you've landed on a desert island and it switches into survival mode. It does three very powerful things to try to keep you alive. Sadly all three are the direct opposite of what you want to happen to lose weight:

1) Your body makes you hungry and sends out signals to make you eat (this alone will make you miserable and ruin most diets);

2) It uses up lean muscle and stores fat (when it thinks it's starving, the body 'dumps' the part of you that needs the most fuel to sustain it – lean muscle);

3) It slows down your metabolism, so you need less and less food and can't seem to lose weight no matter how little you eat.

You cannot afford to have your body fighting you when you are trying to lose weight. So, whatever you do, ditch any diet advice you can remember that told you to eat less, let alone do more. The Harcombe Diet is going to deliver the promises on the back cover, so, get ready to lose weight quickly, easily and healthily and keep it off.

Part One

For Starters

1

What is The Harcombe Diet?

I don't know anyone who wants to be fat and yet 70% of the USA population is overweight and one third obese. Why?

To be slim, we are told that we just need to "eat less and/or do more." Quite specifically, the advice is:

"To lose 1lb of fat you need to create a deficit of 3,500 calories." (This is known as "the calorie theory").

So, why don't we just follow the advice? Why on earth do we have an obesity problem, let alone an epidemic, when we so desperately want to be slim?

The Harcombe Diet is the result of twenty years of research trying to answer this question. The journey has taken me through thermodynamics, peanuts under Bunsen burners and more obesity journals than hot dinners. The conclusions have been staggering and The Harcombe Diet has incorporated all the findings:

1) The calorie theory is wrong.

I blow apart every aspect of the calorie theory in my book *The Obesity Epidemic: What caused it? How can we stop it?* (2010). One pound does not even equal 3,500 calories – not even close. We will *not* lose a pound each and every time we create a deficit of any fixed number of calories and nor will we gain a pound for a repeated surplus.

Every obesity journal I have reviewed from the past 100 years proves this (although they don't always conclude the same). I cannot find one single occasion when this 3,500 formula holds, let alone each and every time. I have also written to five government and two obesity organisations (in my home country, the UK) and none can provide evidence for this formula. Yet all continue to repeat it as a slogan in their literature and spoken advice and it has become folklore on the internet and in gyms world-wide.

2) The current diet advice is actually the *cause* of the obesity epidemic; never will it be the cure.

As recently as 1977, public health advice changed from "carbs are fattening" to "base your meals on carbs" and "avoid (saturated) fat". This U-Turn in dietary advice has had catastrophic consequences. It is no coincidence that obesity has gone up multiples since we changed our diet advice. Public health authorities need to reverse this advice as soon as possible. Until they do, we need to ignore it.

3) The only way to lose weight is to work with your body – never against it.

If you try to eat less, your body fights you every step of the way, as the introduction set out. You are going to discover the power of your body working with you, and not against you, as you lose weight.

4) Weight gain and loss depends on what we eat, what we eat with what and how often we eat. In no way is it as simplistic as just how much we eat. Weight gain and loss also depends far more on carbs consumed, than calories, or fat, consumed.

This doesn't mean that we can't eat carbs. It means that we need to use everything we know about carbs, insulin, how the body uses food for energy and how the body stores fat, so that we can eat the right carbs, in the right way, and still lose weight.

5) Overweight people are not greedy, weak-willed or in need of a psychiatrist. They are victims of the wrong advice.

Seven in ten people are overweight. I do not believe that 70% of the population has a psychological issue with food. I do believe that the majority of people have at least one physical reason (one of three common conditions) driving their food consumption. I also believe that the avoidance of hunger is such a fundamental human instinct that telling people to eat less will make them eat more.

2

How is it different to other diets?

1) **It works.** I set out to understand why we had an obesity epidemic and to design a diet that would eliminate hunger and food cravings. I did not set out to design a diet that would lose people 17lbs in five days and yet, at the time of going to print, this is the record for Phase 1. As a bonus, the most common themes in the endless testimonials are: "I'm not hungry"; "My cravings have disappeared"; "I feel great"; "I've got more energy than I've ever known" and "This is the last diet I will ever need".

2) **It fundamentally rejects the calorie theory**, upon which 99% of diets are based.

The other 1% of diets are the very low carb Atkins and Co. These will work, if you can stick to them, but I don't think that many people need to go to this extreme to lose weight. If you want to lose weight, gain health and enjoy a great variety of food, you may like this diet.

The 99% will *not* work, and we have a century's worth of obesity journals to prove this. (You would also not be reading this book if calorie counting did work). One definition of madness is to do the same thing again and again and to expect a different result. To go on a calorie restricted diet, is therefore, mad.

The Harcombe Diet is so simple; for centuries it was accepted as the *only* way to eat. It is based on the principle that nature knows best. Not the United States Department of Agriculture, not food manufacturers – nature.

On this diet, we eat only real food – food in the form that nature intends us to eat it. We eat this natural food in sufficient quantities to nourish our body and at regular intervals to give the body no reason to store fat. We don't eat processed food – food in the form that food manufacturers intend us to eat it.

3) **The new and unique contribution of The Harcombe Diet** is the discovery that there are three very common medical conditions that cause insatiable food cravings and that these conditions, in turn, are caused by eating less.

The Harcombe Diet has been carefully designed to be the perfect diet to overcome all three conditions. These conditions, by the way, come with a whole range of other, nasty, symptoms. So, if you just want to lose weight, this book will tell you how. If you want to get rid of things as wide ranging as dandruff or waking up at 4am – this book could help you with way more than your waistline.

So here's a summary of what the diet means for you:

- Because it rejects the calorie theory, it does not try to get you to eat less, so quantities are unlimited;
- Because it rejects the calorie theory, it does not try to get you to do more, so exercise is optional;
- Because it is based on working with, not against, your body, you eat regular, healthy meals and your body stops storing food and fat (you also start to feel healthy and much better about yourself);
- Because it's a lifestyle change, it gives you three simple rules, to lose weight and stay slim for life.

I've been asked by the media – if you don't agree with the "Eat less, do more" advice – what do you agree with? My answer is "Eat better and do whatever you like".

I've also been asked – is the diet low carb or low-fat and the answer is neither. It is real food – carbs and fats – in whatever quantities you want – just not at the same meal. All will be explained...

Zoë Harcombe

Author, Nutritionist & Obesity Researcher (BMI 21)

3

What can you eat?

Phase 1 gives you a five-day plan for life, which can lose you up to 17lbs any time you need a quick fix. You can eat meat, fish, eggs, vegetables and salads (not potatoes and mushrooms), Natural Live Yoghurt (NLY) and some brown rice. Other than the brown rice, quantities are *unlimited*. You can have bacon and eggs for breakfast; steak for lunch and curry for dinner.

Phase 2 should be followed for as long as you want to lose weight. (The tips you'll pick up in Phase 2 will stay with you for life). You will be able to eat any real food: steak; pork chops; lamb shank; fish; seafood; cheese; (wholemeal) pasta; (wholemeal) bread; fruit and baked potatoes. You will be able to enjoy (red) wine and dark chocolate, on occasions. Dinner could be a salmon starter, pork chops and vegetables for the main course, strawberries and cream for dessert and a cheese platter – if you've got room.

Phase 1 and Phase 2 are set out for what I have called "Flexis" and "Planners". Flexis don't want a prescriptive diet – they want a list of 'do's' and 'don'ts' and a list of suggested meals and they then get on and do their flexi plan. Planners want to know what to have on Monday for breakfast and Tuesday for lunch and they are quite happy for someone to have planned this all out for them. This book caters for both Flexis and Planners.

Phase 3 takes the principles of Phase 2 and adds in all that you need to know to 'cheat'. 'Cheating' then lets you enjoy literally any food, or drink, without putting on weight.

If you have little to lose and just want to pick up some great tips for eating well when it's no hassle and 'getting away with it' for the rest of the time – you'll get all of this from Phase 3.

Part Two

Main Course

4

Phase 1

WHAT you can eat and drink in Phase 1

Meat:

As much fresh, unprocessed, meat, as you want. This can be white meat and birds (chicken, duck, goose, guinea fowl, pheasant, quail, rabbit and turkey), or, red meat (bacon, beef, fresh ham, lamb, pork, veal and venison). Please check all ingredients, as packaged and tinned meats usually have sugars and other processed things in them. Buying from the (local) butcher, or supermarket meat counter, will be safest.

Fish:

As much fresh or tinned fish as you want – no smoked fish (because it feeds one of the conditions we're going to learn about). This can include white fish like cod, haddock, halibut, plaice, turbot and whiting. It can include oily fish like anchovies, mackerel, pilchards, salmon, tuna, and trout. It can include shellfish and seafood like clams, crab, lobster, mussels, oysters and prawns. Check that the tinned fish that has no added ingredients other than oil or salt. You can cook fish in olive oil, or butter, or steam, bake or grill it.

Eggs:

As many eggs as you want (chicken, duck or any others you like). These can also be cooked with butter.

Brown rice or oats:

You can have up to 50 grams (dry weight – before cooking) of whole-grain brown rice per day, *or* brown rice cereal, *or* brown rice pasta, *or* porridge oats. If you are vegetarian, (or vegan), you can have up to 150 grams (dry weight) of these foods, per day, to make sure that you get enough to eat. You don't have to eat the rice or porridge, but it will give you useful energy.

Salads and Vegetables:

You can have as many salads and vegetables as you want, except mushrooms and potatoes (these are not good for two of the conditions we are going to learn about).

I've listed all that I can think of below:

- Salad stuff – alfalfa, bean sprouts, beetroot, celery, chicory, cress, cucumber, endive, all types of lettuce, radish, rocket, spring onions, water cress and a couple of fruits – olives and tomatoes.

- Vegetables – artichoke, asparagus, aubergine/eggplant, bamboo shoots, broccoli, Brussels sprouts, Bok choy, cabbage, carrots, cauliflower, celeriac, chillies, courgettes/zucchini, fennel, garlic, green/French beans, kale, leek, mange tout, marrow, okra, onions, parsnip, peas, peppers (any colour), pumpkin, salsify, shallots, spinach, squashes, swede, turnip, water chestnuts.

- Any herbs, spices or seasoning – basil, bay leaves, caraway, cardamom, chervil, chives, cinnamon, cloves, coriander, cumin, dill, fennel, ginger, marjoram, mint, nutmeg, oregano, paprika, parsley, pepper, rosemary, saffron, sage, salt, tarragon, thyme, turmeric.

Natural Live (Bio) Yoghurt (NLY):

This might seem a bit 'girly' until you taste full fat, creamy, Greek style yoghurt, that just happens to have this 'live' stuff in it and then you'll be hooked. It's great for snacks and for making Phase 1 feel indulgent.

Tofu:

This is a vegetarian protein alternative, which is fine in Phase 1, provided that it doesn't contain added ingredients. This may not have you salivating, but it is really tasty stir-fried, so give it a go.

<u>Drinks:</u>

You can drink as much bottled water (still or sparkling) or tap water as you like during Phase 1. You can drink herbal teas, decaffeinated tea and decaffeinated coffee.

You must not drink alcohol, fruit juices, soft drinks, canned drinks (even sugar-free drinks), caffeinated products or milk. So, just to be clear, you can't have milk in tea or coffee during Phase 1.

<u>Note:</u>

Don't worry about mixing fats and carbs in Phase 1. Phase 1 gets the results, without adding in this Rule, which you will come across in Phase 2.

Don't eat anything that is not on the list above during Phase 1. No fruit, no wheat or grains (other than the brown rice/oat options listed), no white rice, no sugar, no cakes, no biscuits, no confectionery, no cheese, no pickled or processed foods. Don't eat anything to which you are allergic – obviously.

HOW long is Phase 1?

Phase 1 lasts for just five days. Why five days? Any food that you have eaten passes through your body in 3-4 days, so this gets rid of any processed foods and foods that have been causing you problems. Also, this strict part of the diet needs to be short enough for you to stick to it, but long enough to have an effect.

You can continue Phase 1 beyond five days if you have a lot of weight to lose and find it easy to stick to. This is the fastest weight loss programme I have come across, so you may be happy to put up with a restricted menu to lose weight fast. Phase 2 adds more foods for variety and nutrients and the weight loss continues to be good, so it's up to you when you move on to the next phase.

WHEN do you eat?

All the foods allowed in Phase 1 can be eaten whenever you want. It is best to get into the habit of eating three main meals a day, with snacks in between only if you are genuinely hungry.

HOW much do you eat?

As much as you want of everything on the 'allowed' list – only the brown rice/oat options are limited. You really can have a large plate of bacon and eggs for breakfast and you can have as much meat, fish, salad and vegetables as you can eat for main meals.

If you need to snack between your three main meals then you can have cold meats, hard-boiled eggs, celery sticks, raw carrots, Natural Live Yoghurt (NLY) or a tin of tuna – whatever it takes to keep hunger away.

WHY does Phase 1 work?

There are three very common medical conditions that cause food cravings and two of the three cause severe water retention. We learn more about these conditions in the next chapter (definitions are in the Glossary). All you need to know for now is that Phase 1 has been scientifically designed to be the perfect diet for zapping these three conditions. Phase 1 is low carb, but not to halitosis levels. You will lose pounds, feel less bloated, and quite likely clear up a lot of other health problems along the way and all without slowing your metabolism or feeling hungry.

The small print

Just a word of caution – you may get some quite nasty withdrawal symptoms in Phase 1. You are going 'cold-turkey' on sugar and caffeine, two potentially addictive substances, and you may get some quite bad headaches if you've effectively been an addict. Taking whatever you normally take for headaches should help.

Phase 1 Meal Suggestions for Flexis

Below are some meal options for Phase 1. Recipes for all of these menu suggestions, and lots more, can be found in *The Harcombe Diet: The Recipe Book.*

Breakfasts:

- Bacon & eggs;
- Scrambled eggs (no milk) – cooked in butter and flavoured with herbs, salt and pepper as desired;
- Plain or ham Omelette (no milk) – cooked in butter and flavoured with salt and pepper as desired;
- Natural Live Yoghurt (NLY);
- 50 grams brown rice cereal. You should be able to find this in normal supermarkets – Kallo® is one brand. (It is surprisingly OK dry);
- 50 grams porridge oats – just add boiling water and stir to the consistency you like.

Main meals (lunch/dinner):

- Any amount of meat & salad/vegetables: e.g.

    - Roast leg of lamb with rosemary & vegetables;
    - Roast chicken with garlic or lemon & vegetables;
    - Pork or lamb chops with herbs & vegetables;
    - Strips of beef or chicken & stir-fry vegetables.

- Any amount of fish/seafood & salad/vegetables: e.g.

    - Salad or salmon Niçoise (fish steak or tinned fish with hard-boiled egg(s), anchovies and green beans on a large plate of salads);
    - Mixed fish platter (chunks of cod, halibut, salmon – whatever is available) & salad/vegetables.

- Any amount of eggs & salad/vegetables: e.g.

  - Omelette & salad;

  - Egg and/or cold meat salad.

- Brown rice dishes: e.g.

  - Paella (seafood & chopped vegetables stir-fried with the brown rice allowance);

  - Curry & brown rice (chicken, beef, veggie curry – your usual favourite, but only using meat, fish, vegetables, herbs and spices allowed in Phase 1);

  - Stuffed tomatoes or peppers (cook the rice, add some cooked chopped vegetables and put this in a large tomato or pepper and bake in a medium oven for 20-30 minutes);

  - Home-made kebabs on brown rice (chunks of meat, fish and/or aubergines/eggplant, courgettes/zucchini, peppers etc);

  - Brown rice with stir-fried vegetables and/or stir-fried strips of meat.

- Vegetarian dishes: e.g.

  - Tofu & vegetables in home-made tomato sauce;

  - Tofu & stir-fry vegetables.

- Starters: e.g.

  - Asparagus in butter;

  - A selection of soups.

- Desserts – Just Natural Live Yoghurt for Phase 1.

Phase 1 – 5 day plan – for Planners

This 5-day plan is just to give you an example for Phase 1. Please remember that, other than the brown rice/oats, quantities are unlimited.

This plan does separate fats and carbs, but you don't need to do this in Phase 1. The shaded lines below are fat meals and the non-shaded lines are carb meals. Replace any meal that you don't like with any other breakfast or main meal from Chapter 4. Have the same breakfast and main meals every day, if this works for you.

DAY 1:

Breakfast	Bacon & eggs
Lunch	Salmon steak(s) with a selection of vegetables and a large side salad; Natural Live Yoghurt (NLY)
Dinner	Vegetables (not potatoes) stir-fried in olive oil with 50 grams brown rice

DAY 2:

Breakfast	50 grams brown rice cereal – no milk
Lunch	Salade Niçoise (a tin of tuna, or a tuna steak, on a bed of salads. Hard-boiled eggs, olives and anchovies are optional); NLY
Dinner	Real meat (steak, pork chops or lamb etc) with any amount of vegetables & salad

DAY 3:

Breakfast	Plain or ham omelette (2-3 eggs, knob of butter, ½ teaspoon mixed herbs, ground black pepper, chopped ham (optional) – whisk the eggs until fluffy, add the herbs and pepper, melt the butter in an omelette pan and add the eggs (and ham), cook slowly until it becomes firm. If you stir the mixture you will end up with scrambled eggs – see Day 5)
Lunch	Chicken and/or beef strips stir-fried in olive oil with vegetables; NLY
Dinner	Stuffed peppers – (boil 50 grams brown rice, stir-fry chopped, mixed, vegetables in olive oil and then mix the rice & vegetables and fill a deseeded pepper shell. Bake in a medium oven for 20-30 minutes, until the pepper is soft to a fork touch)

DAY 4:

Breakfast	50 grams porridge oats with water (literally put dry oats in a bowl and pour boiling water on top to the consistency you like)
Lunch	Chef's salad (a large mix of salads, grated carrots, grated beetroot, fennel etc – be really creative, with cold cuts of meat and/or hard-boiled eggs); NLY
Dinner	A large whole fish, like trout or mackerel, with plenty of vegetables and salad (or real meat, like Day 2)

DAY 5:

Breakfast	Scrambled eggs (no toast) or soft boiled eggs with Crudité 'soldiers'
Lunch	Roast or grilled chicken & salad and/or vegetables; NLY
Dinner	50 grams dry weight rice pasta in home-made tomato sauce (stir-fry an onion and a clove of garlic in olive oil, add a tin of tomatoes, 2 teaspoons of basil and ground black pepper and simmer the sauce until the rice pasta is ready)

You may drink as much bottled water (still or sparkling) or tap water as you like during Phase 1. You can drink herbal teas, decaffeinated tea and coffee (no milk).

You may have any soup, (or other starter), which uses only foods allowed in Phase 1. Lots of options can be found in *"The Harcombe Diet: The Recipe Book."*

You may have any vegetables and salads, except mushrooms and potatoes, in Phase 1.

If you need to snack you can have NLY; Crudités (sticks of carrots, celery, peppers etc); hard-boiled eggs; extra meat and/or fish.

5

Phase 2

WHAT you can eat and drink in Phase 2

Phase 2 has just three rules. Learn to love them as much as your favourite TV channel, as this is the secret to being fit, not fat, and staying there. The three rules are:

1) Don't eat processed foods;

2) Don't eat fats and carbs at the same meal;

3) Don't eat any foods that you currently crave.

RULE NUMBER 1

Don't eat processed foods

The single simplest thing you can do to get to your ideal weight and stay there is to eat real food and absolutely nothing processed. Real food is food in the form as provided by nature. Oranges grow on trees, cartons of orange juice don't. Baked potatoes come out of the ground, chips don't. Cows graze in a field, Peperamis® don't – you get the idea.

The most commonly found processed food is sugar (sucrose) and this is particularly important to avoid, as it has no nutritional value. It gives you energy, (calories), but nothing else that you need. Avoid sugar in any form – white or brown. Anything with syrup in the title or "*ose*" at the end is usually sugar e.g. sucrose, glucose syrup, corn syrup, maltose, fructose, dextrose etc. Watch out – sugar is in cakes, biscuits, confectionery, almost every cereal, most bread, ready meals, many crisps, most desserts, many types of yoghurt and even tins of kidney beans and chickpeas.

Below is a list to summarise the real foods, which should be eating and the processed foods, which you want to avoid:

DO EAT – REAL FOOD	DON'T EAT – PROCESSED FOOD
Meat: Any pure meat with no food processing e.g. pork chops, steak, lamb joints, chicken, carvery meat etc. Best sources will be the local butcher or the fresh meat counter in the grocery store. The butcher may have sausages with only meat and meat products (nothing else added) – these are fine	Processed meats e.g. burgers, meat sticks, normal sausages etc Tinned meats often have ingredients added – check the label Sliced packaged meats usually have sugars, like dextrose, added
Fish & Seafood: Any fish or seafood from the fishmongers or the fresh fish counter/aisle in the grocery store. Most tinned fish is OK – tuna, salmon, sardines – anything in just oil, brine or plain tomatoes is fine	Processed fish – fish fingers, fish in batter, fish in breadcrumbs (contains white bread and sugar). Any microwave meals (fish or meat) invariably have sugars or other processed ingredients
Eggs & Dairy: Any eggs Any real milk, cheese, yoghurt, butter, cream	Flavoured yoghurts, processed cheese sticks & slices, margarine and manufactured spreads

DO EAT – REAL FOOD	DON'T EAT – PROCESSED FOOD
Fruit & Vegetables: Any whole fruits (eating the skins where edible) Baked potatoes with the skins on Any other vegetables	Fruit juices or dried fruits e.g. raisins Chips, crisps Vegetable juices, Vegetable crisps
Grains: Brown rice Wholemeal pasta Wholemeal flour Wholemeal bread (with no sugar, glucose syrup, treacle or other processed ingredients)	White rice White pasta White flour White bread, or any bread with sugar or sugar substances in it
Sugar: Any sugar found naturally in whole food: fruit sugar in the whole fruit (fructose); milk sugar in milk (lactose)	Any sugar – white or brown; Any 'ose' added to products – e.g. maltose, dextrose, sucrose, fructose; treacle; honey etc.
Drinks: Water, milk, any herbal teas, Decaf tea & coffee	Canned drinks (sugared or sweetened), fruit juice

RULE NUMBER 2

Don't eat fat and carbs at the same meal

We need a quick fact box here – just to help with knowing your fats from your carbs...

> Fact Box: All food is carbohydrate, protein or fat – or, invariably, a combination of two or three of these. Fruit is mostly carbohydrate, with some protein and usually no fat. Meat is protein and fat and has no carbohydrate. Protein is in everything, from lettuce to bread to fish, so we could classify food into fat/protein and carb/protein, but it's easier to just drop the word protein. The two really interesting food groups are carbohydrates and fats. Why are they so interesting? Because one causes the body to release a substance called insulin and the other doesn't. More later.

... and how to remember this...

> Fact Box: The best way to remember the difference between a carbohydrate and a fat is that a fat comes from something with a face. All meat and fish were animals – with faces. Eggs, butter and cheese all come from animals – with faces. The exceptions are oils like sunflower oil and olive oil, but don't worry about these – the only fats you need to think about are the ones from the faces.
>
> Carbs come from the ground and trees: fruits, grains, potatoes and so on. If it isn't an oil and it doesn't come from a face, it's a carb.

Rule 2 is – eat either fat at a meal, or eat carbohydrate, but don't mix the two. The exception is that salads and vegetables have a low carbohydrate content and can, therefore, be eaten with either fat or carbohydrate meals. So your meals should be 'fat' meals (e.g. meat, fish, cheese, eggs) with salad and/or vegetables *or* 'carb' meals (e.g. brown rice, wholemeal pasta, baked potato) with salad and/or vegetables.

As a general rule, coloured and/or root vegetables, (e.g. butternut squash, carrots, parsnips etc), have a higher carb content, so go easy on these with fat meals. Potatoes (normal and sweet potatoes) should *not* be seen as vegetables – think of them as staple carbs, which form the basis of a carb meal.

Three other foods to be careful of are nuts, seeds and avocado. Nature naturally separates foods into fat/protein or carb/protein (isn't that interesting?), but these are key exceptions:

- 100 grams of peanuts, as an example, have 25 grams of carbohydrate and 51 grams of fat;
- Sunflower seeds have 20 grams of carbohydrate and 51 grams of fat; and
- Avocado has 9 grams of carbohydrate and 15 grams of fat. These are real and nutritious foods, but not great for weight loss.

Finally, milk and yoghurt are the interesting animal foods. Meat and fish are totally carb free. Eggs, cheese and cream are virtually carb free, but milk and yoghurt, both low-fat and real, have approximately five grams of carbohydrate per 100 grams. This is still very low in carbohydrate, but go easy on the lattés and NLY – especially between meals.

On the following page there is a useful list to show which foods can be eaten as a fat meal and which can be eaten as a carb meal and which can be eaten with either. If you're allergic to anything in here, e.g. fish, then obviously don't eat it.

FAT MEALS	CARB MEALS
Any unprocessed meat –bacon, beef, chicken, duck, goose, guinea fowl, ham, lamb, pheasant, pork, quail, rabbit, turkey, veal, venison	All **Fruit** **Whole-grains** – brown rice, brown pasta, brown rice pasta, couscous, 100% wholemeal bread, quinoa, millet etc.
Any unprocessed fish – cod, haddock, halibut, mackerel, plaice, pilchards, salmon, seafood, trout, tuna, whiting etc. Includes tinned fish in only oil, salt and/or water	**Wholemeal cereal** – porridge oats, Brown rice cereal, Shredded Wheat®, other sugar-free cereal
Eggs – Chicken, duck etc.	**Beans & Pulses** – lentils, broad beans, kidney beans, chickpeas etc.
Dairy Products – Cheese, milk, butter, cream, yoghurt (ideally Natural Live Yoghurt)	Baked **Potatoes** in their skins

EAT WITH EITHER A FAT OR A CARB MEAL

Salads – alfalfa, bean sprouts, beetroot, celery, chicory, cress, cucumber, endive, all types of lettuce, radish, rocket, spring onions etc.

Vegetables – artichoke, asparagus, aubergine/eggplant, bamboo shoots, broccoli, Brussels sprouts, cabbage, carrot, cauliflower, celeriac, chillies, courgettes/zucchini, garlic, green beans, kale, leek, mange tout, marrow, okra, onions, parsnip, peas, peppers (any colour), pumpkin, salsify, shallots, spinach, squashes, swede, turnip, water chestnuts etc.

Tofu/Quorn – Vegetarian protein alternatives

Certain **Fruits** – olives, tomatoes & berries

Low-fat dairy products – milk, cottage cheese & yoghurt

Herbs, Spices & Seasoning – basil, chives, coriander, cumin, dill, fennel, mint, oregano, paprika, parsley, pepper, rosemary, sage, salt, thyme etc. Olive oil for cooking.

How to use this list:

1) You can eat anything on the fat list with anything on the 'eat with either' list. You can eat anything on the carb list with anything on the 'eat with either' list.

2) You should *not* eat anything on the fat and carb lists at the same meal.

3) Generally, when fat is removed from a product something else needs to be put back in to replace it. The exception to this is with animal fat products, where fat can be removed and nothing needs to be put back in its place. So, where there are low-fat alternatives to standard products like milk and yoghurt, these can be eaten with carb meals. This lets us have skimmed milk with cereals and low-fat cottage cheese with baked potatoes, for example.

4) The fruits on the 'eat with either' list, (olives, tomatoes and berries), have a carb content more like vegetables, than fruit and so they can be eaten with either fat meals or carb meals. (Don't eat olives by the bucket load, with carb meals, however, as olives also have a reasonable fat content). These fruits give the diet some great menu options, as it means you can have berries and low-fat yoghurt after a carb meal. It also means that you can have tomato pasta sauces, as well as using tomatoes and olives in meat and fish dishes.

5) Try to leave three to four hours between a fat meal and a carb meal, because this is the time that food normally takes to be digested. You should achieve this naturally by having three meals a day. If you are eating snacks (not ideal), have carb snacks between carb meals and fat snacks between fat meals (the menu plan at the back gives you an illustration).

RULE NUMBER 3

Don't eat foods that you currently crave

We need three more fact boxes here – just to give you simple definitions for three very common medical conditions, which cause food cravings and stop you losing weight. These conditions are Candida, Food Intolerance and Hypoglycaemia.

Fact Box: **Candida** – is a yeast, which lives in all of us, and is normally kept under control by our immune system and other bacteria in our body. It usually lives in the digestive system. Candida has no useful purpose. If it stays in balance, it causes no harm. If it multiplies out of control, it can create havoc with every aspect of our health.

Fact Box: **Food Intolerance** – means, quite simply, not being able to tolerate a particular food. Food Intolerance develops when you have too much of a food, too often, and your body just gets to the point where it can't cope with that food any longer. Food Intolerance can make a person feel really unwell.

Fact Box: **Hypoglycaemia** – is literally a Greek translation from "*hypo*" meaning 'under', "*glykis*" meaning 'sweet' and "*emia*" meaning 'in the blood together'. The three bits all put together mean low blood 'sugar' (glucose). Hypoglycaemia describes the state the body is in if your blood glucose levels are too low. When your blood glucose levels are too low, this is potentially life threatening and your body will try to get you to eat.

The clue to which condition (or all three) that you have is what you crave...

If you have **Candida** (classic symptoms are dandruff, athlete's foot and a white coating in your mouth when you wake up), you are likely to crave bread, pizza, beer, cereal, biscuits, sweets, pickled foods and blue cheese. You will need to avoid these and limit all carbs, even fruit, in Phase 2.

If you have **Food Intolerance**, you will crave the thing(s) to which you are intolerant. The most common food intolerances are the things that we eat every day – wheat, milk and sugar being the main culprits. Be honest, whichever food(s) you really feel you couldn't live without are the ones you need to give up. You won't have to give them up forever, but just until you've lost weight and got your immune system back in good shape. Then you'll be able to re-introduce them (you just won't be able to have too much of them and too often).

Classic symptoms of **Hypoglycaemia** are: waking at 4am hungry and possibly with night sweats; an 11am and 4pm 'dip' during the day, where you feel irritable, hungry and unable to make a decision; and general cravings for sweets and sweet foods. These foods then give you an instant sugar rush, followed by an energy dip and cravings for more sweet foods. If you have Hypoglycaemia, limit all carbs in Phase 2 and have as many fat meals as possible. Have no more than 1-2 pieces of fruit per day during Phase 2 and go for lower sugar fruits like apples, pears, citrus fruits and berries. Avoid tropical fruits, like bananas, melons and so on.

If you have more than one condition, you will need to follow the advice for all the conditions that affect you. This will restrict the foods that you can eat, but this is only until your immune system recovers and your body can tolerate your problem foods again. You are not giving up these foods for ever.

Time for some science:

We need a few fact boxes here – to share the minimum you need to know about your blood glucose level, insulin, and glycogen and why insulin is called the fattening hormone:

Fact Box: **Glucose** is the primary fuel needed by the human body. (It is the petrol in our car in effect).

Fact Box: **Blood Glucose Level** – Our normal levels of blood glucose are around 65-100 mg/dl (milligrams per decilitre of blood). When our blood glucose level stays above this level the impact is serious and can even be fatal.
Without knowing the medical detail of high, low and normal blood glucose levels, you will probably be familiar with the effects. When you eat any carbohydrate, you may experience a surge of energy as the glucose floods into your blood stream – literally a sugar high. Low blood glucose (**Hypoglycaemia**) is what you may have experienced, often late morning, late afternoon, or soon after a sugar high, when you feel irritable, hungry, have difficulty concentrating and may even have slightly shaky hands.
The body's blood glucose level is crucial to our well-being and it is also crucial to our desire to lose weight.

Fact Box: The **Pancreas** is an organ in the body located below and behind the stomach. Its main functions are a) to produce the hormones insulin and glucagon and b) to produce digestive enzymes to help digest (break down) the food that we eat. In a Type 1 Diabetic, the pancreas doesn't work and this person needs to inject insulin, sometimes several times a day.

Fact Box: **Insulin** is a hormone produced by the pancreas. When we eat a carbohydrate our body converts this into glucose and so our **Blood Glucose Level** rises. This is dangerous for the human body, so the pancreas ensures that insulin is released to convert the excess glucose to **Glycogen**, to return our **Blood Glucose Level** to normal.

Fact Box: **Glycogen** is the storage form of glucose found in the liver and muscles. The liver has the capacity to store approximately 100 grams of glycogen. The muscles have the capacity to store between 250-400 grams of glycogen, depending on your muscle mass, physical condition and regular carbohydrate intake. Liver glycogen supplies energy for the entire body. Muscle glycogen only supplies energy to muscles. Each molecule of glycogen, stored within the liver and muscles, is bound to approximately four molecules of water. Hence, for each gram of glycogen stored, approximately four grams of water are also stored.

Putting all this together, we come up with the key fact:

Fact Box: Every time you eat a carbohydrate, your body decides how much of the energy consumed is needed immediately and how much should be stored for future needs. As your **Blood Glucose Level** rises, **Insulin** is released from the **Pancreas** and this insulin converts some of the **Glucose** to **Glycogen**. If all the glycogen storage areas are full, insulin will convert the excess to fatty tissue. **This is why insulin has been called the fattening hormone.**

HOW long is Phase 2?

Follow Phase 2 for as long as you want to lose weight. If you have approximately 15-20lbs, or less, to lose then you could easily lose 5-7lb in Phase 1 and you may only need to follow Phase 2 for a couple more weeks. If you have a lot of weight to lose then you can be free from hunger and food cravings throughout Phase 2 and you will lose weight while eating healthy, natural foods, which your body will thank you for.

WHEN do you eat?

Eat whenever you want, in Phase 2, but try to get into the habit of eating three substantial meals a day and only snacking in between if you are genuinely hungry.

Now that you know that insulin is the fattening hormone, you know that the fewer times you raise your blood glucose level during the day, the better. If you snack on low-fat/high carb foods, you are causing your body to release insulin on a more regular basis and this won't help you to lose weight.

Just as insulin facilitates fat storage, so it prevents fat burning. Eating a carb 'injects' glucose and insulin into the blood stream and this has been shown to diminish the level of fatty acids almost immediately. Until the carb, glucose and insulin arrived, the fatty acids were being used for fuel. You want to optimise the hours during which your body is using fat for fuel and not glucose – another reason not to snack.

HOW much do you eat?

Eat what you need. However, just because quantities are unlimited doesn't mean that you're training for an eating contest. Don't go hungry, but don't go mad either. One of the many reasons that this diet works so well is that you will find it almost impossible to overeat. The body has a natural appetite mechanism when given only real food.

WHY does Phase 2 work?

The rationale behind Phase 2 is really simple and powerful:

Rule 1 – Don't eat processed foods

This is because when you eat processed foods your body is highly likely to release too much insulin (e.g. if you drink orange juice, your body thinks you have eaten several oranges and pumps out enough insulin to mop up lots of oranges). We must stop this happening for two key reasons:

1) As insulin is the fattening hormone we want our bodies to release the right amount of insulin to mop up the food we

have actually eaten, not too much, so that the extra is stored as fat. If we eat the whole orange or whole grains, i.e. the whole food every time, our bodies should release the right amount of insulin.

2) If we end up with too much insulin, after eating something, our blood glucose level will be low, which will make us crave food to get our blood glucose level back to normal. So, we will have cravings for food – especially processed foods – which is what has made us eat junk and put on weight in the first place.

Processed foods are 'empty calories'. They give us calories, i.e. energy/fuel, but they don't give us as many vitamins and minerals (nutrients) as we could get from eating the same number of calories from real food. If we don't get the nutrients we need, we will crave foods to find other ways of getting these nutrients. If we eat a varied diet of real food – meat, fish, eggs, dairy products, vegetables, salad and fruit – we will be more likely to get the nutrients we need and our body won't need to crave things. If we eat microwave meals, cakes and biscuits and so on, we are going to crave more food to get the nutrients.

Rule 2 – Don't eat fats and carbohydrates at the same meal

The easiest substance for the body to get energy from is carbohydrate. So, if your body spots that you've eaten a carb it says "Thank you very much – I'll use that for my immediate energy needs and I'll store any fat with it for later on". The double whammy is that the body needs insulin to store fat, and it is only carbohydrates that cause insulin to be released. So, your body can only store that fat, for later on, when you have eaten a carbohydrate.

As an example, if you eat a bacon butty the body will take the bread and tomato sauce carbs for immediate energy and store the bacon and butter for later on. *And* the body is only able to store the fat because insulin has been released and this only happened because of the bread and tomato sauce. The 'great' American diet is based on mixing fats and carbs: hot dogs with buns; burgers and chips; pizza with meat and/or cheese topping – no wonder we're overweight.

If you eat carbohydrate, and no fat, the body uses the carbs for energy and there is no fat to store. If you eat fat, and no carbohydrate, your body has to use the fat for energy and it has to work a bit harder to do this (which is good news for you, because it naturally uses up more energy). As we don't want to facilitate fat storage, we don't want to eat these two food groups at the same time.

Rule 3 – Don't eat foods that you currently crave

You crave the foods that feed any of the three conditions, from which you may be suffering, because Candida, Food Intolerance and Hypoglycaemia all lead to unbelievable food cravings. To lose weight comfortably, you have to stop the cravings. To stop the cravings you have to get these three conditions back under control.

Phase 2 Meal Suggestions for Flexis

Below are some meal options for Phase 2. Recipes for all of these menu suggestions, and lots more, can be found in *The Harcombe Diet: The Recipe Book*.

You can have a fat meal or a carb meal whenever you like. The more fat meals you have, the quicker you will lose weight (carbs and insulin really are the secret to weight loss). However, do balance this with the nutrients and menu variety that come with good carbs and enjoy carb meals as part of Phase 2.

With all of the following, don't forget to add in Rule 3 and avoid the food(s) that you crave... So, limit fruit to 1-2 pieces a day for Candida and Hypoglycaemia and have rice pasta, instead of wheat pasta, and no bread, if you have wheat intolerance.

Breakfasts – fat meals

- Bacon & eggs (no ketchup or brown sauce);
- Kippers/smoked haddock;

- Scrambled eggs;
- Plain, ham or cheese omelette;
- Natural Live Yoghurt (NLY);
- Cooking options for fat breakfasts include grilling, poaching, steaming, baking or frying in butter or vegetable oil.

Breakfasts – carb meals

- Fruit platter (optional low-fat NLY);
- Shredded Wheat® & skimmed milk (with a sliced banana – optional);
- Brown rice cereal (with skimmed milk or great on its own, as it stays crunchy);
- 100% porridge oats with water, or skimmed milk;
- Sugar-free muesli with water, or skimmed milk;
- Wholemeal bread & marmite.

Main Meals – Starters – fat meals

- Prawn cocktail;
- Tomatoes & mozzarella;
- Asparagus in butter;
- Salmon & cream cheese;
- A selection of soups.

Main Meals – Starters – carb meals

- Char grilled vegetables with olive oil or balsamic;
- Vegetable kebabs;
- Melon selection;
- Fruit salad;
- A selection of soups.

Main Meals – Main Courses – fat meals

- Any amount of meat & salad/vegetables: e.g.
    - Roast leg of lamb with rosemary & vegetables;

- Roast chicken with garlic or lemon & vegetables;
- Pork or lamb chops with herbs & vegetables;
- Strips of beef or chicken & stir-fry vegetables.
- Ham, egg, cold meat salad (Chef's salad);

- Any amount of fish/seafood & salad/vegetables: e.g.
  - Tuna or salmon Niçoise (fish steak or tinned fish with hard-boiled egg(s), anchovies & green beans on a large plate of salads);
  - Mixed fish platter (chunks of cod, halibut, salmon – whatever is available) & salad/vegetables.

- Any amount of eggs/cheese & salad/vegetables: e.g.
  - Omelette (with or without cheese) & salad;
  - Four cheese salad;
  - Cauliflower cheese and/or cheesy leeks;
  - Egg & asparagus bake;
  - Egg and/or cold meat salad.

- Vegetarian dishes: e.g.
  - Tofu & vegetables in home-made tomato sauce;
  - Quorn & vegetables in home-made tomato sauce;
  - Tofu or Quorn & stir-fry vegetables.

Main Meals – Main Courses – carb meals

- Brown rice & stir-fry vegetables;
- Quinoa with stir-fry vegetables;
- Wholemeal pasta & tomato sauce;
- Wholemeal spaghetti & tomato sauce;
- Vegetarian chilli & brown rice;
- Couscous & char grilled vegetables;
- Vegetarian curry & brown rice;

- Baked potato & salad and/or very low-fat cottage cheese and/or ratatouille;
- Roasted vegetables with pine nuts & Parmesan cheese;
- Stuffed tomatoes and/or stuffed peppers.

Main Meals – Desserts – fat meals

- Strawberries (or any berries) & yoghurt or cream;
- Sugar-free ice cream;
- Natural Live Yoghurt;
- Greek Yoghurt (can be full fat with a fat meal);
- Cheese selection (no crackers or grapes).

Main Meals – Desserts – carb meals

- Any berries with very low-fat yoghurt (e.g. strawberries, raspberries, blackberries etc).

A note here on fruit: fruit salad is the obvious carb dessert, but don't go for this. Eat fruit alone or before any other food. Fruit digests in less than half an hour. Some foods take about four hours. If you eat fruit after steak, for example, the fruit gets stuck behind the meat in the digestive tract and your stomach will bloat. The only exception to this is berries – you can eat strawberries, raspberries etc at the end of a meal, as relative to other fruits, they are very high in water content, high in dietary fibre and low in sugar. Strawberries for example are 92% water vs. a banana at 74%. Blackberries have five times the dietary fibre of an apple (per 100 grams) and dietary fibre passes through the stomach undigested and more slowly. Raspberries have half the sugar content of apples.

Snacks – fat options

- Cheese;
- Hard-boiled eggs;
- Natural Live Yoghurt;
- Cold cuts of meat.

Snacks – either

- Crudités (sticks of carrots, celery, peppers etc).

Snacks – carb options

- Sugar-free cereal bars – ideally wheat-free also. Health food shops have a reasonable selection;
- Sugar-free oat biscuits (ingredients of oats, oil & salt only);
- Fruit (ideally lower sugar fruits like apples, pears, citrus fruits and berries);
- Rice cakes (high Glycaemic Index, so avoid these if you are very carb sensitive).

Easy Lunches for Work – fat meals

- Tinned tuna/salmon with salad in a lunch box;
- Cold meat (chicken/turkey/beef/ham) with salad;
- Any fat leftovers from dinner the night before;
- Frittata – cold omelette.

Easy Lunches for Work – carb meals

- Brown bread sandwich with anything low-fat e.g. salad, hummus, cottage cheese;
- The 'national dish' of Israel: wholemeal pita bread stuffed with falafel and salad;
- Brown rice salad – cold brown rice with chopped salad ingredients;
- Any carb leftovers from dinner the night before;
- Baked potato & salad and/or low-fat cottage cheese;
- Fruit platter.

A note here on wheat intolerance: you may well find wholemeal pita bread OK, even if normal bread causes bloating and other problems.

Phase 2 – 7-day plan – for Planners

This example 7-day plan assumes that you have Candida, wheat Food Intolerance and Hypoglycaemia and excludes the foods that you should avoid for each of these. This plan assumes that you do *not* have dairy intolerance and are, therefore, fine with milk and cheese. Please remember that, other than the pieces of fruit specified, quantities are unlimited.

The shaded lines below are fat meals and the non-shaded lines are carb meals. You can swap in any fat or carb meal, from this chapter, whenever you like, to add variety and to avoid something that you may not like. You can also add any carb starters or desserts from this chapter to carb meals and add any fat starters or desserts to fat meals. Many more options can be found in *The Harcombe Diet: The Recipe Book.*

It is ideal to *avoid snacks*, and get used to eating three large meals a day, but Day 1 sets out the best snacks to go for, if you really need something and it sorts the 'not mixing' timescales for you. A fat snack (in the shaded areas) can be NLY or a decaff cappuccino/latté. A carb snack can be 1-2 pieces of lower sugar fruits or 1-2 oat biscuits.

You may drink as much water (still or sparkling) as you like. You can drink herbal teas, decaffeinated tea and coffee. There are some notes on caffeine and alcohol at the end of this 7-day plan.

DAY 1:

Breakfast	Bacon & eggs
AM snack	NLY or decaff. cappuccino/latté
Lunch	Salade Niçoise
PM Snack	1-2 pieces of fruit or 1-2 oat biscuits
Dinner	Vegetarian curry & brown rice

DAY 2:

| Breakfast | Porridge with water (or skimmed milk) |
| Lunch | Brown rice salad (cold rice from night before with chopped peppers, spring onions, cucumber etc) |

| Dinner | Roast chicken with vegetables & salad; cheese platter (no grapes or crackers) |

DAY 3:

| Breakfast | NLY |
| Lunch | Chef's salad |

| Dinner | Brown rice & stir-fry vegetables (& tofu – optional) |

DAY 4:

| Breakfast | Brown rice cereal |
| Lunch | Baked potato & low-fat cottage cheese or low-fat NLY or ratatouille |

| Dinner | Pork or lamb chops or salmon steaks with vegetables & salad |

DAY 5

| Breakfast | Scrambled eggs |
| Lunch | Baked, poached, grilled, fried or steamed fish & vegetables |

| Dinner | Rice pasta in home-made tomato sauce (see recipe from Phase 1 Day 5) |

DAY 6

| Breakfast | Porridge with water (or skimmed milk) |
| Lunch | Char grilled vegetables & brown rice |

| Dinner | Steak & mixed grill or a large fish like trout or mackerel with vegetables & salad |

DAY 7

| Breakfast | Plain or ham omelette (with milk and cheese, if no dairy intolerance) |
| Lunch | Roast lamb, pork, beef or chicken with vegetables & salad |

| Dinner | Vegetarian chilli & brown rice |

Caffeine, Chocolate and Alcohol...

It is ideal in Phase 2 to avoid caffeine, chocolate and alcohol, but a man's got to enjoy life. So here is how to 'cheat' in Phase 2 to make it work for you:

Caffeine: If you just can't face the thought of starting the day without an espresso or regular coffee or tea, then have one. However:

- Try not to go over one, maximum two, cup(s) a day. Caffeine stimulates the production of insulin in a similar way to carb consumption, so you can't afford to have much, before weight loss will be impacted;
- Have your early morning coffee with a carb, rather than a fat, breakfast, as the caffeine will raise your blood glucose level and you don't want that insulin in your body looking for a fat breakfast to store;
- Caffeine will give you a short term high followed by an energy low, so have a strategy for getting your blood glucose level back to normal. One guy I worked with had his espresso as soon as he woke up and then had his cereal after showering, so that the breakfast naturally raised his blood glucose level back to normal after the caffeine high.

Chocolate: This is my favourite food, so I'm happy to help others find a way of enjoying chocolate while still losing weight. However:

- If you must have chocolate in Phase 2, it has to be real chocolate – at least 70% cocoa and ideally 85% cocoa (or higher). Milk 'chocolate' is primarily sugar and milk powder and it's not OK in Phase 2;
- You still shouldn't go mad even with real chocolate (save that until Phase 3). Have an occasional square or two – best at the end of a fat meal, as a dessert.

Alcohol: The other thing that some people just can't do without is a glass of wine with dinner:

- Go for red wine, rather than white. There is some debate as to the health properties of red wine and the claims are likely exaggerated. However, red wine does contain resveratrol and antioxidants and these could provide health benefits;
- If you have white wine, go for dry to limit the sweetness that you consume;
- Try to have no more than one glass a day with your main meal and ideally not every day.

Match day: There are some days when you are going to want to drink rather more than a glass of wine! It may be match day, or your birthday, or just Saturday night out. Here are the tips for how to do this:

- Accept that you are not going to lose weight on this day, but aim not to put any on instead;
- Follow Phase 2 rules for as much of the day as you can (right up until the evening if it's a night out);
- Have a fat meal (e.g. bacon and eggs) a couple of hours before the drinking starts – this will 'line' your stomach and help keep your blood glucose level stable;
- Alcohol impairs the operation of a hormone (glucagon), which naturally raises your blood glucose level. This is why drinking gives you the munchies (and why you only ever fancy a kebab on the way home from the pub/club). Try to wait for a bowl of porridge when you get home instead.

Maximising weight loss in Phase 2: The less you 'cheat', the more weight you'll lose, simple as that. You may want to be quite strict in Phase 2, to lose weight quickly, and then 'cheat' with Phase 3, when you are at your target weight. You may want to cheat more along the way and accept that the weight loss will be slower, but at least you can have your favourite things as you go along. It's entirely up to you.

A note about exercise

As promised on the cover, you do not need to exercise to lose weight. Remember that other diets are trying to create a calorie deficit (eat less/do more) and this diet is based on the principle that this calorie theory is fundamentally incorrect.

Don't get me wrong, exercise is a great thing to do – it will build muscle, make you feel better, give your heart a workout, keep the dog happy. It delivers the three S's: Stamina, Suppleness and Strength. If you have a lot of weight to lose, I would highly recommend exercise to develop lean tissue, as you lose weight, to get a great shape as an end result.

There are many good reasons to exercise, but because you think it will make you lose weight is not one of them. Can one thought help convince you? You can eat in one minute what can take an hour to burn off. The importance of *not* eating something in the first place is incomparable with the idea that you can eat what you want and then use up the fuel.

This begs the question – surely if I do both – eat well (not eat less) *and* exercise, this can only be a good thing. The answer is – it depends on whether or not your activity levels drive your eating or the other way round.

Exercise can increase your desire for food (fuel) in two ways – both continuously and at the time:

1) Exercise raises your Basal Metabolic Rate (BMR), which means you need more fuel (calories) continuously, just to run your basic body functions;

2) Exercise is likely to make you hungry at the time. If you go somewhere in the car, you need to put more petrol in the tank. Your body will demand just the same when you have finished your gym session (well trained bodies demand the fuel in advance).

If you can manage the additional demand for food that exercise will produce, without eating the wrong things, because you have 'run out of petrol', then exercise should do no harm. If, however, you find yourself eating muffins at the gym café, or continually craving carbs to replenish your glycogen stores, then exercise may in fact hinder your weight loss.

If your eating drives your activity levels, on the other hand, this can only be a good thing. I believe that the precursor of doing more is eating better. I think that it is as likely that people are sedentary because they are obese, as they are obese because they are sedentary. I think that a switch to eating only real food, in unlimited quantities, is likely to give people the energy and desire to be more active. This is a great side effect of The Harcombe Diet and one to be embraced. (Interestingly, we tend to get the direction of causation right when we insult people. We tend to say "fat people are lazy", rather than "lazy people are fat". The former supports my view that people are sedentary because they are obese).

If you try to use exercise as the starting point for change, you run the risk of unhelpfully increasing your demand for fuel and for carbs particularly. The starting point for change must be to eat well (i.e. real food in nourishing quantities). Then you can do as much as you have the energy to do and you are then in an eat well/feel well/do more/eat well cycle.

The Harcombe Diet is all about working with your body, so do this with exercise as well as with food. Listen to your body and let it tell you what it wants to do. If you do exercise because you feel you ought to and not because you enjoy it, don't bother (or find something more fun). If you enjoy exercise, don't stop!

6

Phase 3

This chapter is the secret of how to have your cake and eat it. This is about eating as much as you can get away with, without putting on weight. It will take a bit of trial and error, but, once you've got it, you'll never look back.

Move onto Phase 3 when you are at what we call your 'natural weight'. This is the weight that you can maintain easily – going above it takes some overeating and going below it only happens when you are ill or under stress. Some men call this their 'fighting weight' – it's what you feel good at, but can also stay at without too much effort.

WHAT can you eat and drink/not eat or drink?

The three rules from Phase 2 should still form the basis of your eating in Phase 3. These really are your top tips for life long healthy eating.

The difference with Phase 3 is that you can also eat what you want *almost* when you want. This is called 'cheating'. The key thing is to make sure that you don't start putting weight back on and here is how you do this:

1) Don't 'cheat' too much;
2) Don't 'cheat' too often;
3) Be alert and stay in control.

Number 1 says don't 'cheat' too much – eat a confectionery bar if you want one, but don't eat ten. Eat a dessert if you want one, but don't eat the bread sticks while you're waiting for your starter. Rule Number 1 is, therefore, about the *quantity* of the processed foods that you eat.

Number 2 says don't 'cheat' too often. Have a dessert for a special occasion, but just not every day. Eat that confectionery bar if you want to, but not every day. Number 2 is, therefore, about the *frequency* with which you eat processed foods. Try to stick to the rules in Phase 2 as often as possible and then only cheat when you really fancy something.

Number 3, is about you having the knowledge and the skills to control your cravings and, therefore, to control your eating and your weight. Get to know what works for you. You may get it wrong the first time and you may find that cravings return. Don't panic. Go back to Phase 2 for however long it takes to get back in control.

To learn from the experience ask yourself some questions – Were you cheating too much (quantity)? Were you cheating too often (frequency)? You were probably more than half aware that you were starting to become quite attached to a particular food or foods and, therefore, you should have cut back earlier as this was the first sign of cravings. Be really honest with yourself next time and as soon as you think you *need* something rather than *want* something, avoid that food totally, for at least five days.

Top tips for becoming a master of cheating

The basics are all you need – don't cheat too much, don't cheat too often and be alert and stay in control. However, if you want to become a gold medallist at cheating, here are the top tips...

Tip 1 – Cheat all at once

If you want a pizza, eat a pizza, but don't keep eating one or two slices throughout the day. Remember, you are trying to minimise the number of times your pancreas releases insulin.

Tip 2 – Eat as few ingredients as possible

The fewer processed ingredients you can attack your body with the better. If you have a packet of crisps, pick the one that has just potatoes and vegetable oil (you don't even need salt). There are some packets of crisps that have more than 100 ingredients in them – steer well clear of these.

If you want ice cream then try Haagen-Dazs® vanilla, which has (in order) fresh cream, skimmed milk, sugar, egg yolk and natural vanilla flavouring and tastes as good as ice cream can possibly get. Don't pick the carton with more ingredients than you can recognise let alone remember.

Tip 3 – Have a strategy for getting your blood glucose level back to normal

If you eat a processed food, your body will almost certainly release too much insulin and this will make your blood glucose level fall lower than before you ate the substance. Your body will then demand food to get your blood glucose level back to normal. This is the time when you are most at risk of craving another processed food. So, anticipate that this will happen and have something healthy to hand when you feel your blood glucose level drop. This can be a piece of fruit or an oat biscuit – any whole food that will get your blood glucose level back to normal naturally.

Tip 4 – Don't eat your normal meal AND cheat

If you are going to have a bag of kettle chips for lunch then make that your lunch. Don't have your steak and salad as well, as your body will just store the fat in the steak when you eat the kettle chip carbs.

Tip 5 – Don't waste cheating

If you are going out for dinner don't start on the nuts and bread sticks before dinner – you know you'll eat them all as soon as you start, so don't even have one. Save your cheating for the real food and enjoy something really special from the menu instead.

Tip 6 – Don't forget that insulin is the fattening hormone

Carbohydrates stimulate the production of insulin, the fattening hormone, but so do caffeine and sweeteners. You may like to return to full caffeine coffee and cola in Phase 3, but this must be counted as cheating. If this is really how you want to use your cheating then do so. Cheating connoisseurs never forget that the key to cheating is to minimise the production of insulin.

Tip 7 – Have exactly what you want

If you want a pint of your favourite lager, don't settle for a low carb beer instead. You'll only have the low carb beer and then still want the lager, so just have it.

Tip 8 – Just because you can cheat doesn't mean you have to

This diet lets you eat every real food on the planet – meat, fish, eggs, dairy products, fruits, salads, vegetables, whole grains. You will not miss out on anything by not eating processed foods so, if you don't have any urge to 'cheat', then don't.

Part Three

Dessert (optional)

7

The three conditions

Of all the things that I discovered, in approximately twenty years of research, this is one of the most interesting findings. Having come across the three very common medical conditions and all the books describing how they cause food cravings, I analysed the causes of the conditions and the most likely cause of all three is trying to follow a calorie-reduced diet. (The fact boxes defining the three conditions are on page 28).

When we try to eat less/cut calories, the following three things happen:

1) We increase the proportion of carbohydrate in our diet. Fat has approximately nine calories per gram while carbohydrate has four, so people trying to lose weight choose carbs over fats every time and thereby increase the proportion of carbohydrate in their diet.

   If this doesn't happen automatically, public health diet advice directs us to do this – "base your meals on starchy foods", "eat more fruit and vegetables", "eat less saturated fat" – all advice is, directly or indirectly, to eat more carbs.

2) We reduce the variety of food eaten. We tend to go for the regular favourites that give us 'the biggest bang for the buck' (the most food for the fewest calories). We probably have a set breakfast – our toast, or cereal, or muffin on the way to the office every day. We likely have a set lunch also – a sandwich, bag of crisps and/or a cereal bar. We may vary the evening meal a bit more, but it is still likely to have the same ingredients in it and always more carbs than fats.

3) We weaken our immune systems. This happens because:

a) We are not eating as much fuel (calories) as our body needs;
b) We have cut back on fats, which are essential for our immune system; and

c) We develop nutritional deficiencies by not eating enough calories and fats and by eating a limited variety of foods (and not least if we are still eating our share of the USA average 400 empty calories of sugar a day).

Candida, Food Intolerance and Hypoglycaemia are caused by a variety of things, ranging from diet to modern medication (e.g. antibiotics and steroids). All three, however, are fundamentally caused by:

1) Consuming a high carbohydrate diet;
2) Eating the same things every day; and
3) Having a weakened immune system.

i.e. the diet composition and nutritional changes that occur when we try to eat less.

So, how did you most likely get these three conditions? By trying to follow any 'normal' (calorie restricted) diet, which drove you down the path of more carbohydrates and more processed food.

How can you make sure they don't come back? Avoiding the medication mentioned (antibiotics, steroids, hormones etc) is helpful, but, by far the most important thing is to never try to follow 'eat less' advice again.

8

"The Viagra Principle"

If this isn't a principle, it should be. It should describe the circumstance when you get something 'for free' when you fix another thing. The well known effect of Viagra was discovered as a side effect to a drug for hyper tension and high blood pressure. It was only when the testers didn't want to return their tablets, that the drug company realised they'd hit a different jackpot.

"The Viagra Principle" applies with this diet: Because Candida, Food Intolerance and Hypoglycaemia cause so many different health problems, when you get them under control you will be so chuffed at how many other things clear up at the same time.

Here are some of the most common symptoms of each condition – which you can expect to get rid of when you follow The Harcombe Diet:

Symptoms exclusive to **Candida** are a coated tongue; athlete's foot; dandruff and other fungal infections. Oh, and hair loss – if that interests you.

The following symptoms are common with both **Candida** and **Food Intolerance**, which is why, so often, people with food cravings and weight problems are suffering from both conditions:

Physical symptoms include: constipation; diarrhoea; bloating; indigestion; gas; heartburn; headaches; dizziness; blurred vision; flushed cheeks; feeling 'spaced out'; quick sugar 'highs' followed by fatigue; waking in the early hours and not being able to get back to sleep; abnormal cravings for sweet foods/bread/alcohol and/or caffeine; muscle aches and dry skin.

Mood Symptoms include: anxiety; depression; irritability; lethargy; memory problems; loss of concentration; moodiness; nightmares; mental 'sluggishness' and "get up and go" has got up and gone.

Hypoglycaemia, in common with the other two conditions, can also cause headaches; dizziness; blurred vision; feeling 'spaced out' and all the mood symptoms listed.

The key problems with Hypoglycaemia, however, are all those related to the blood glucose level. Sufferers will experience the following: hunger between meals; irritability before meals; feeling faint/shaky when food is not eaten; irregular pulse before and after eating; headaches late morning and late afternoon; waking in the early hours and not being able to get back to sleep; abnormal cravings for sweets or caffeine; eating sweets only increases hunger; excessive appetite; instant sugar 'high' followed by fatigue.

All of these can be dramatically improved, if not eliminated altogether, on The Harcombe Diet. How's that for a Viagra Principle?

9

Fitness and nutrition

If you run or cycle long distances, this is how to optimise your performance while managing your weight. Please note that eating for fitness and eating for weight loss are not always compatible. It is possible (and better for weight, if not performance) to fuel on fats, rather than carbs, even for extreme physical challenges. However, eating for fitness for most people, in most cases, means consuming a regular supply of carbs; eating for weight loss is the opposite. Your weight loss may actually suffer if you are determined to train hard.

The key principles remain the ones from Phase 2…

1) Don't eat processed foods;
2) Don't eat fats and carbohydrates at the same meal;
3) Don't eat any foods that you currently crave.

… then you add these three tips, for fitness training:

1) The single biggest tip is to get to know *your* body. It is different to every other body out there, so you've got to find out what works for you: How well can *you* store carbs? At what point does *your* body run out of glycogen? How long before this happens do *you* need to eat something? What food works best for *you* before, during and after a training session? Keeping a food and training diary can really help you to understand this.

2) Optimal fitness is then all about being able to a) consume, b) store and c) use energy optimally:

a) Serious exercisers need to *consume* good carbs regularly (wholemeal bread, wholemeal pasta, brown rice, baked potatoes, starchy fruits and vegetables etc). Sports nutritionists advise eating carbs six times a day, leading up to a race/training session.

b) Glycogen, remember, is the form in which glucose (energy) is *stored* in the liver and muscles. There are two key aspects to glycogen storage:

i) The body can only store glycogen for 24 hours so the 24 hours before a race/training session are the most critical time to load those good carbs into the storage room. Anything put in the 'glycogen storage area' and *not* used within 24 hours will be converted to fat;

ii) You can train your body to get better at storing glycogen. Glycogen storage depends on muscle mass, physical condition and regular carbohydrate intake. So, you can build muscle, train and eat good carbs regularly to optimise your ability to store energy. You should be able to store approximately 100 grams of glycogen in the liver and 250-400 grams in the muscles.

c) Glycogen stored is used up within approximately two and a half hours of intense exercise. To *use energy* optimally you need to know when your own storage room empties and you need to eat a banana or whole grain energy bar 20-30 minutes before your own storage is going to run out. Never let the 'carb larder' run empty.

3) Don't forget breathing and water. The unit of energy in the body is called ATP (Adenosine TriPhosphate). The macro nutrients (carbs, proteins and fats) are converted by the body into glucose and ultimately into this 'energy currency'. For sprinters this happens anaerobically (without oxygen). For distance athletes, this happens aerobically (with oxygen). The by-products of aerobic metabolism are carbon dioxide, which we breathe out, and water.

So, runners need a continual supply of a) fuel (e.g. glycogen stored in the body, carbs recently eaten), b) oxygen (work on achieving a comfortable and relaxed breathing style), and c) water (as soon as a person loses just 2.5% of their body weight from water loss, they lose 25% of their physical and mental abilities).

10

Eating out and losing weight

The key principle, when eating out, is that you will rarely find good carbs. Hence, main meals will invariably need to be fat meals when away from home.

Eating out, here are some headlines for what to go for in the likely favourites:

Coffee Shops – many coffee shops stock 70% dark chocolate next to the till. You could do a lot worse, for a lunch on the run, than a large decaf cappuccino/latté and a bar of dark chocolate, for a 'fat meal'. You'll be getting protein, calcium and iron and enough energy to get you through to the next meal.

If you've got more time, or are going back to the office, most of the coffee shop chains have tuna or chicken salads in the chiller cabinets. Avoid the potatoes, white pasta and sugary salad dressings, but the salad and fish/meat itself will be fine.

Chinese restaurants are great for The Harcombe Diet. Choose meat, fish, seafood and vegetable dishes, but avoid the sweet and sour sauces, as these have sugar in them. Go for the spicy sauces instead, as these are rarely sweetened. Skip the rice, noodles and fortune cookie carbs. Eat with chopsticks and then any sauce is likely to stay on the plate. Desserts are not a feature of oriental meals, so there will be no temptation after the main courses. A green tea will aid digestion to finish the meal (please note that green tea contains caffeine).

European cuisine can work really well. Here are some examples:

With French food you will be spoiled for choice – meat, fish, seafood, (Salade Niçoise), cheese and eggs are found in abundance in France (hence why the French are so slim as a nation). Skip the white French bread and Gratin Dauphinois (potatoes in cheese).

Greek food is also ideal – Greek salad, stuffed olives, meat kebabs, fish dishes. Greek restaurants do some amazing aubergine/eggplant, olive oil and cheese dishes (great fat meals).

Finally, Italian – skip the white bread and pasta and go for the tomatoes and mozzarella, baked fish, plain meat or meat in sauces and all the Italian vegetables and mixed salads that go with this. If you fancy a dessert, go for Italian creamy ice cream, over sorbet every time. Real ice cream will be fat/cream based. Sorbet is virtually pure sugar.

On **Holiday** and in **Hotels**, you may be able to have a carb breakfast – if you can find porridge oats, Shredded Wheat®, fresh fruit and very low-fat yoghurt, for example. You can also have an omelette or "English breakfast" as a fat meal, without bread, baked beans, red or brown sauces, or any carbs.

For main meals, you should find an excellent choice of (local) fresh produce for fat meals – meat, fish, cheese, vegetables and salads. You can usually find omelettes on the menu. If you like fish, go for the 'catch of the day'. Local meat specialities are likely to contain only real ingredients (even if in a casserole type of dish).

Indian cuisine is also great for The Harcombe Diet. Go for any number of meat, fish, seafood and vegetable dishes and avoid all carbs – naan bread, white rice, poppadoms, onion bhajis etc. Dry dishes, like Tandoori Chicken or King Prawns, are especially healthy. All the Tikka dishes, with the spicy yoghurt dressing, are great fat meals.

Japanese and Thai restaurants can be even better for your diet than Chinese. Their cuisine tends to be 'drier' – less in the way of rich sauces and more in the way of hot stuff like wasabi (Japan) and chillies (Thai). You'll be looking for meat, fish, seafood and vegetable dishes again and you should find everything from raw fish (Japanese) to spicy stir-fry beef (Thai).

USA local 'cuisine' generally is not great for healthy eating and it's even worse if you're a vegetarian. (California is an exception – this is such a healthy American state that you'll even be able to find brown rice and good carbs). Across the States, avoid the absolute mass of take-away and processed food and go for the steak houses and salad bars. Baked potatoes are quite commonly found, so you can have some carb meals (ask for low-fat sour cream and salad to go with your spud). Otherwise, look for International cuisines when you eat out. I've eaten Japanese, Chinese, Indian and all sorts in the USA, but rarely eaten 'American'.

Vegetarians always have a more limited choice and are much better off with Asian cuisines than Western (many Asian countries avoid particular animal consumption for religious reasons). Veggies should be able to get Tofu/soya bean and vegetable dishes in Indian and/or oriental restaurants. In the worst case, go for plain white rice, vegetable spring rolls and other vegetable dishes for an OK 'carb' meal. This isn't ideal, but it's a good example of how, sometimes, you need to go for the least worst option when eating out and learn 'damage limitation'.

Vegetarian restaurants can give anyone access to great carb meals. Invariably good vegetarian chefs use whole grains, so you may get whole wheat burgers, couscous, quinoa and some new carb options to try. Student cities and cosmopolitan cities are particularly good for vegetarian whole foods. You've got more chance of finding vegetarian restaurants in California and New York than Alaska and Wyoming.

11

Cholesterol, fats and health

The purpose of this chapter is to explain why The Harcombe Diet does not worry one iota about any fat or cholesterol, found in real food, which you eat.

Time for a bit more science

Let us gather a few facts first: What is cholesterol? What is fat? What is the difference between saturated and unsaturated fat?

> Fact Box: **Cholesterol** is a waxy substance found in the cell membranes and transported around the body in the blood stream. Chemically speaking, cholesterol is an alcohol (hence the "*ol*" at the end). It is more commonly called a fat, as thinking of it as an alcohol is not helpful. Far from being the bad substance that propaganda would have us believe, cholesterol is absolutely vital for life.

Cholesterol is so critical to the human body (you would die instantly without it), that the body does not leave it to chance that you could get such a life vital substance from food. Your body makes cholesterol. One of the major reasons why humans need to sleep is so that the body has time to make cholesterol and to do repair work around the body. Here are just some of the vital functions that cholesterol performs:

- Cholesterol, like fat, is a major building block in the regeneration of cells. Hair and finger nails are obvious cells, which are continually being replaced, but virtually all cells are replaced many times over during our lifetimes.
- Cholesterol is vital for the ongoing maintenance of all cells in the body – allowing nutrients to pass into the cells and waste products out. It also enables the proper digestion of fats and the accompanying management of waste products.
- Cholesterol is crucial for brain function and nerve transmission (which is why some of the most serious side

effects of statins – drugs that stop the body making cholesterol – are memory loss and other mental problems).
- Cholesterol is also essential for our immune system; it works with sunshine to make vitamin D; it maintains hormone production (including sex hormones – another side effect of statins can be loss of sex drive).

Reading this you should rightly be questioning why most doctors seem so intent on lowering the cholesterol level of every human – men especially. If I tell you that one statin alone, Lipitor®, is worth over $12 billion, you may understand.

It is a common misconception that there is such a thing as LDL (bad) cholesterol and HDL (good) cholesterol. Cholesterol is not water soluble, so it cannot be transported freely in the blood-stream to where it is needed. It needs to be carried somehow and it is carried in things called lipoproteins (short hand for the words lipids and proteins). LDL stands for Low Density Lipoprotein and HDL stands for High Density Lipoprotein. LDL carries cholesterol from the liver out around the body to do its cell repair and other jobs. HDL carries cholesterol, which has been used by the body's cells, back to the liver for re-use (re-cycling in effect). Neither LDL nor HDL is cholesterol – they are carriers of cholesterol – and neither is 'bad' or 'good'.

Fact Box: **Fat** is also a waxy substance found in the cell membranes and transported around the body in the blood stream. As with cholesterol, fat consumption is crucial for our well-being. Every cell of our body depends on adequate fat intake.

Saturated fats are the most stable fats (this is merely a statement about chemical structure). They have all available carbon bonds filled with (i.e. saturated with) hydrogen.

Monounsaturated fats have one double bond in the form of two carbon atoms 'double-bonded' to each other and, therefore, lack two hydrogen atoms.

Polyunsaturated fats have two or more pairs of double bonds and, therefore, lack four or more hydrogen atoms.

There are four types of fat – one should not exist. The three fats in the previous fact box are real and essential for health. These are the only fats that we care about on The Harcombe Diet – the ones found naturally in real foods.

The fourth fat is the one made by man, manufactured by hydrogenating (adding hydrogen atoms to) vegetable oils, to make them solid at room temperature. These have been banned in Denmark, Switzerland and some American States and, frankly, should be banned world-wide. Numerous studies have shown them to have serious, likely carcinogenic (cancer causing) properties and they have no place in a healthy diet. They are typically found in margarine, low-fat spreads and many processed foods – all things we naturally avoid on The Harcombe Diet.

Every real food, which contains fat, has all three real fats in it – only the proportions vary. Hence meat, fish, eggs, dairy foods, nuts, seeds and oils all contain saturated *and* monounsaturated *and* polyunsaturated fat. Coconuts are one of the rare foods that are mostly saturated fat. Olive oil is mostly monounsaturated fat and sunflower seeds are mostly polyunsaturated fat. You may also be interested to know that the main fat in beef, pork, eggs and even lard is *monounsaturated* fat, not saturated fat. People trying to get you to avoid red meat, eggs and natural fats kept that one quiet, did they not?

The key point is that all real foods, with a fat content, contain all three fats. None of these fats is better or worse than the others – they are all needed and they are all found in real food in the 'right' proportions for our survival. Dieticians would have us believe that saturated fat is trying to kill us and unsaturated fat is trying to save us. So, 39% of your steak or pork chop is trying to kill you and the 61% *unsaturated* fat content is trying to save you? Puh-lease! Do you really think that Mother Nature is trying to kill you?!

"Let them eat butter"!

When we are told to eat less saturated fat, the following are the products that we are told to avoid (the lists from the NHS and the Food Standards Agency are virtually identical):

- Processed foods: Meat products, such as sausages and pies; pastries; cakes; biscuits; savoury snacks; crisps; sweets snacks; chocolate and ice cream.
- Real foods: "Fatty meats", dairy products and that most commonly used food (not) – coconut oil. The dairy devils are listed: cheese, butter, cream, crème fraîche and "full fat" milk (oh come on guys, whole milk is still only 3.5% fat).

So, let's agree the battleground. The fundamental principle of The Harcombe Diet is to "Eat food in the form that nature intends us to eat it." On this basis I am in 100% agreement with public health messages to avoid the processed foods listed above. However, this is because processed food should be avoided *per se*. None of these foods need be avoided for any real fat, which they may contain, saturated or otherwise. The main ingredients in the processed foods above are refined carbohydrates (primarily sugar and white flour) and, quite likely, man made fats, which no human should ingest. If any of these foods contain small quantities of real foods like butter and meat, these will be the absolute healthiest part of the product by a margin!

Common sense tells us that the longer we have been eating a particular food and the closer we eat it in the form that nature intended, the less likelihood there can be that the food is bad for us.

We have been eating fat and cholesterol, found naturally in animals and animal by-products, since man first walked the planet (*"Australopithecus Lucy"* is believed to be the first 'dude' (ape/man – whatever) – dating back approximately 3,500,000 years). If anything in animals were bad for us, let alone responsible for a killer disease, evolution tells us that we would have either a) died out or b) evolved to not need the 'fatal' substance. As there is no evidence of either a or b, common sense alone tells us that we are quite safe eating animals and animal products. (History tells us that we evolved as omnivores and would have consumed any limited berries, nuts and vegetation in the natural environment. However, the fact that we consumed any animals that we could catch cannot be in doubt).

Here's another way of looking at it: if we started eating animals 24 hours ago, agriculture (large scale access to carbohydrates) developed four minutes ago and sugar consumption has increased twenty fold in the last five seconds. I wonder which food is more likely to be responsible for any modern disease...

Now, if you want, an area of compromise could be to eat meat without worry and to eat low-fat dairy products instead of the real versions (and, presumably to avoid cheese, as there is no decent low-fat alternative to this). This is your choice and indeed I advise low-fat dairy products if you're having a carb meal. However, that advice is to keep fats and carbs separate (for all the reasons we have seen). When you have a fat meal, you should eat real foods. Dairy products contain the fat soluble vitamins, A, D, E and K and this means they need to be delivered in fat to be absorbed by the body. How sensible of nature to put fat soluble vitamins in fats and how stupid of humans to remove the fat and thereby the delivery mechanism.

As a final thought, nature warns us off foods that are bad for us by making them bitter and 'distasteful' in some way. Can someone please explain bacon therefore?!

12

Did you know?

Asparagus: Ever wondered why your wee smells funny after eating asparagus? This was first investigated in 1891. There are a number of chemicals in asparagus, which are not found in any other food. They are metabolised (broken down) by the body and they produce some interesting and quite smelly by-products (one of which is methyl mercaptan, as an example). Studies have shown that not everyone is able to produce these by-products and some people produce them, but can't smell them. So, if you can do both, you can be proud of your chemical metabolic mechanism!

Chocolate: The carbohydrate content of chocolate varies inversely to cocoa content. 100 grams of milk chocolate has 54 grams of carbohydrate; 100 grams of 70% cocoa chocolate has 32.5 grams and 100 grams of 85% cocoa chocolate has just 19 grams of carbohydrate – fewer than in an apple.

Constipation: If you ever suffer from constipation, first make sure that you are drinking enough – constipation is invariably due to *insufficient* liquid intake. The next best tip is vitamin C: This water soluble vitamin cannot be stored by the body, so your body will get rid of any excess of vitamin C and take any other waste products with it. You can find your 'poo tolerance level of vitamin C' – the level that results in regular bowel movements without going too far – by trying a 500mg tablet of vitamin C and then, if you need to, increasing the number of tablets each day. You'll work it out!

Drinking with meals: Red wine is the only drink that you should have with meals. Water and other drinks flood your natural digestive juices and stop food being digested effectively. Drink your fluid intake *between* meals, not during.

Fat vs. water loss: The average male is 50-60% water, so you are always going to lose water at the same time as fat. Keeping the maths simple, a 200lb man who loses 100lb is not going to lose 100lb of fat alone and turn into a puddle! A pound of weight is a pound of weight when it comes to the scales, your clothes and how you look. If you are *not* de-hydrated, and weigh less than last week, that weight loss counts.

Milk: This is one of nature's most interesting foods. Strictly speaking milk is for babies, but it is one of the most nutritionally complete foods on the planet and, therefore, common sense says that anyone who can tolerate milk should consume it. We need the enzyme lactase to digest milk and the body produces far less lactase after we reach the age of two. This is why lactose (milk) intolerance is quite common. If you find milk 'disagrees' with you, you are best avoiding it in large quantities. However, most people, even if lactose intolerant, will be able to have a small amount of milk.

Six pack: This is the term used to describe clearly defined abdominal muscles. You've got these already. You just need to get rid of any fat covering them. Forget the gym and sit-ups. Lose weight; aim for a body fat content below 10% and you'll find the male model underneath!

Sugar: provides no nutritional value – no protein, vitamins or minerals – it gives us calories and nothing else. Cutting sugar out of your diet loses you nothing of value – there is always a more nutritious way to get the calories (fuel) that you need.

Water: If you ever feel hungry, try drinking a glass of water. It is estimated that 75% of people are dehydrated much of the time and they are actually 'hungry' for liquid (water), not food. Fruit can be 95% water and even meat can be as high as 75% water, so the body will try to get water in whatever way it can.

Wind: is largely trapped air, so you can take steps to reduce the volume of air inside your digestive system that wants to find a way out. Drinking fizzy drinks puts unnecessary air bubbles inside you and they have to come out in a burp, or at the other end. Talking while you're eating makes you swallow air, (so women should arguably be windier than men!)

Glossary

This Glossary has all the definitions from the Fact Boxes and a couple of other definitions (marked as "New"), which you may find useful.

Blood Glucose Level: Our normal levels of blood glucose are around 65-100 mg/dl (milligrams per decilitre of blood). When our blood glucose level stays above this level the impact is serious and can even be fatal.

Body Mass Index (BMI) (New): This is the measurement that is used to define 'overweight'. It is calculated by taking a person's weight in kilograms and dividing this by their height in metres squared, e.g. our Mr average, with a height of 5'9" and a weight of 172lbs has a BMI of 78kg/(1.75m x 1.75m) = 25.4. This is just in the overweight range.

The guidelines are:

- A BMI of less than 18.5 is considered "*Underweight*";
- A BMI of 18.5 – 24.9 is considered "*Normal*";
- A BMI of 25 – 29.9 is considered "*Overweight*";
- A BMI of 30 or more is considered "*Obese*".

BMI is only a guide. It takes no account of muscle vs. fat for example. Using the BMI scale, many athletes, and almost all rugby or American Football players, are classified as overweight. If you are an athlete or an ex-athlete you will know if you are a solid bloke, or a flabby one needing some attention.

A useful secondary measure to add to BMI is waist measurement. If the BMI scale says that you're overweight or obese, and you have a waist circumference greater than 94cm (37in), don't kid yourself that you're slim. Men with a waist measurement of more than 102cm (40in) are considered to be at high risk of diabetes, stroke and heart disease.

Check your BMI on any BMI calculator on the internet. There is one on www.theharcombediet.com.

A **Calorie (New):** "The amount of energy required to raise the temperature of 1 gram of water from 14.5'c to 15.5'c, at standard atmospheric pressure."

Candida: is a yeast, which lives in all of us, and is normally kept under control by our immune system and other bacteria in our body. It usually lives in the digestive system. Candida has no useful purpose. If it stays in balance, it causes no harm. If it multiplies out of control, it can create havoc with our health.

Carbohydrates: come from the ground and trees. The main carbs are therefore vegetables, fruits, potatoes, grains (rice, wheat, pasta, bread etc). If it isn't an oil and it doesn't come from a face, it's a carb.

Cholesterol: is a waxy substance found in the cell membranes and transported around the body in the blood stream of all animals. It is vital for our health.

Diabetes: is the condition that someone has if their pancreas does not produce any, or enough, insulin to return their blood glucose level back to normal after they have eaten a carbohydrate. Before the drug insulin was developed, Diabetics had to follow a diet with virtually no carbohydrate, to ensure that their blood glucose level stayed within the normal range.

Fats: (i.e. dietary fats) come from something with a face. All meat and fish were animals – with faces. Eggs, butter and cheese all come from animals – with faces. The exceptions are oils like sunflower oil and olive oil, but don't worry about these – the only fats you need to think about are the ones from the faces.

Food: All food is carbohydrate, protein or fat – or a combination of two or three of those. Fruit is mostly carbohydrate, with some protein and virtually no fat. Meat is protein and fat and has no carbohydrate. Protein is in everything, from lettuce to bread to fish, so we could classify food into fat/protein and carb/protein, but it's easier to drop the word protein.

Food Intolerance: means, quite simply, not being able to tolerate a particular food. Food Intolerance develops when you have too much of a food, too often, and your body just gets to the point where it can't cope with that food any longer. Food Intolerance can make a person feel really unwell.

Glucose: is the primary fuel needed by the human body. (It is the petrol in our car in effect).

Glycaemic Index (New): this is the measure of the effect of any food on blood glucose levels over a period of time. Glucose is the purest substance from which the body can get energy. The index uses the impact of pure glucose being consumed as '100' and then measures all other foods against this.

Glycogen: is the storage form of glucose found in the liver and muscles. The liver has the capacity to store approximately 100 grams of glycogen. The muscles have the capacity to store between 250-400 grams of glycogen, depending on your muscle mass, physical condition and regular carbohydrate intake. Liver glycogen supplies energy for the entire body. Muscle glycogen only supplies energy to muscles. Each molecule of glycogen, stored within the liver and muscles, is bound to approximately four molecules of water. Hence, for each gram of glycogen stored, approximately four grams of water are also stored.

Hypoglycaemia: is literally a Greek translation from "hypo" meaning 'under', "glykis" meaning 'sweet' and "emia" meaning 'in the blood together'. The three bits all put together mean low blood sugar (glucose). Hypoglycaemia describes the state the body is in if your blood glucose levels are too low. When your blood glucose levels are too low, this is potentially life threatening and your body will try to get you to eat.

Insulin: is a hormone produced by the pancreas. When we eat a carbohydrate our body converts this into glucose and so the level of glucose in our blood rises. This is life threatening to the human body so the pancreas releases insulin to convert the excess glucose to glycogen, to return our blood glucose level to normal.

Insulin resistance (New): describes the situation where our bodies don't respond properly to the release of insulin. With insulin resistance, eating carbohydrates causes insulin to be released, but the body fails to use this insulin efficiently and, therefore, the carbohydrates get stored as more fat instead, adding to your weight problem further. It has been shown that 92% of people with type 2 Diabetes have insulin resistance. (Type 2 Diabetes is the one developed by older people – not the one that teenagers tend to get very suddenly).

The **Pancreas:** is an organ in the body located below and behind the stomach. Its main functions are a) to produce the hormones insulin and glucagon and b) to produce digestive enzymes to help digest (break down) the food that we eat. In a Type 1 Diabetic, the pancreas doesn't work and this person needs to inject insulin, sometimes several times a day.

Syndrome X (New): is a term used by doctors to group together a number of conditions, which they have often seen together in a patient. They have observed that people with insulin resistance are also highly likely to have: unnatural blood fat levels; unnatural lipoprotein levels; glucose in the blood; high blood pressure and so on. By looking at these conditions together they are able to treat the patient 'holistically' and try to address all the problems together as they are linked – all related to the weight and blood glucose handling mechanism of the patient.

Shopping List

Here is a shopping list for the Phase 1 plan in Chapter 4. This will be enough for one person (unless indicated otherwise), so just double the quantities if you can persuade someone to join you. I have suggested quantities but have more or less to suit your needs:

Eggs: a dozen should be enough, even if you go for all the egg options.

Fish: Salmon – 200g; Tuna – 200g (tinned or fresh); 1 large whole fish (like trout); tin of anchovies (optional for the Salade Niçoise).

Meat: 100g bacon; 250g steak/pork or lamb; 250g chicken or beef for stir-fry; 250g chicken or ham for chef's salad; add another 100g ham if you want this in your omelette; portion of fresh chicken for roasting. (You may like to buy a large whole chicken for Phase 1 and use accordingly).

Salad stuff: 250-500g salad leaves (or 1-2 large iceberg lettuces); 1 cucumber; 1 celery; 1 bunch spring onions; 250g tomatoes (cherry tomatoes are good with salads); 1 fennel; 1 fresh beetroot – include as many salad varieties as you can. 4-6 peppers (to be used in stir-fries and stuffed peppers).

Vegetable selection: aim for approximately 200g (pre-cooked weight) of vegetables for each of the 5-7 times you have a selection of vegetables i.e. 1-1.5 kilos of vegetables in total. E.g. a head of broccoli, 2 courgettes/zucchini, 4 onions, 6 carrots, 2 leeks, small cabbage, small cauliflower, small packet of green beans, small packet of baby sweet corn, anything that you like, in season.

Brown rice cereal – generally comes in a 250g packet.

Porridge oats – not the jumbo oats – just plain oats – the smallest bag is probably 500g.

Brown rice – (short grain tends to be 'nuttier'; long grain tends to be softer). The smallest bag you are likely to find is 500g.

Brown rice pasta (in the gluten free section of the supermarket) – 250g bags are usually available.

Tins of tomatoes – Two 400g tins of chopped tomatoes.

NLY – Five 250g tubs of Natural Live Yogurt should be fine or three 500g tubs. Get more if you think you will need more.

Staples that you will need to get if they aren't at home: black pepper, cloves of garlic, mixed herbs, basil, butter, jar of olives, olive oil.

Also by Zoë Harcombe:

Stop Counting Calories & Start Losing Weight

Let me guess...

You've tried every diet under the sun;
You've lost weight and put it all back on;

The more you diet, the more you crave food;
You have almost given up hope of being and staying slim.

Do you want some good news? It's not your fault.
You are not greedy or weak-willed.
You've just been given totally the wrong advice.

This is the first book to explain why traditional diets are the cause of the current obesity epidemic, not the cure.

It shows that eating less leads to three extremely common physical conditions, which cause overeating.

This book can change your life. The Harcombe Diet® will help you lose weight & keep it off.
There is absolutely nothing to count and you can have unlimited quantities of real food - carbs and fats.

Count Calories and end up a food addict.
Stop Counting Calories & Start Losing Weight!

Published by Columbus Publishing Ltd – 2011

ISBN 978-1-907797-11-8

Also by Zoë Harcombe & Andy Harcombe:

The Harcombe Diet
The Recipe Book

Real food; great taste; optimal health – that's what The Harcombe Diet is all about and here's how to do it.

With over 100 recipes for Phase 1, another 100 for Phase 2 and then just a few seriously special Phase 3 cheats, this is the ultimate diet-recipe book.

You can have burgers, seafood risotto and authentic Indian curry in Phase 1; boeuf bourguignon, mushroom stroganoff and cream berry pudding in Phase 2 and the most sensational dark chocolate mousse in Phase 3.

This features Harcombe friendly versions of the classic dishes – French onion soup, coq au vin, chilli con carne and the classic accompaniments – mayonnaise, chips and cauliflower cheese.

If you want to eat real food, lose weight and gain health – this is a must for your kitchen shelf.

Published by Columbus Publishing Ltd – 2011

ISBN 978-1-907797-07-1

Also by Zoë Harcombe:

The Obesity Epidemic:
What caused it? How can we stop it?

We want to be slim more than anything else in the world,
so why do we have an obesity epidemic?

If the solution is as simple as 'eat less and do more',
why are 90% of today's children facing a fat future?

What if the current diet advice is not right?
What if trying to eat less is making us fatter?
What if everything we thought we knew about dieting is wrong?

This is, in fact, the case.

This book will de-bunk every diet myth there is and
change the course of The Obesity Epidemic.
This is going to be a ground breaking journey, shattering every
preconception about dieting and turning current advice upside down.

Did you know that we did a U-Turn in our diet advice 30 years ago?
Obesity has increased 10 fold since – coincidence or cause?

Discover why we changed our advice and what is stopping us
changing it back; discover the involvement of the food industry in our
weight loss advice; discover how long we have known that eating less
and doing more can never work and discover what will work instead.

There is a way to lose weight and keep it off, but the first thing you
must do is to throw away everything you think you know about
dieting. Because everything you think you know is actually wrong.
The diet advice we are being given, far from being the cure of the
obesity epidemic, is, in fact, the cause.

Published by Columbus Publishing Ltd – 2010

ISBN 978-1-907797-00-2

Index

alcohol 14, 41, 42, 52

ATP (Adenosine TriPhosphate) 55

Australopithecus Lucy 62

avocado 25

Basal Metabolic Rate 43

Blood Glucose 28, 30, 31, 53, 66

BMI 66

caffeine 15, 41, 47, 52, 53

calorie 9, 43, 50

Candida 28, 29, 34, 39, 51, 52, 67

cereal 12, 16, 18, 21, 26, 29, 35, 38, 40, 41, 50

chocolate 10, 41, 56, 64, 73

cholesterol .... iii, 59, 60, 62, 67

coffee 14, 20, 23, 39, 41, 47, 56

constipation 52, 64

cream 10, 22, 26, 35, 37, 46, 57

dandruff 9, 29, 52

Diabetes 66, 67, 69

Eating out .... iii, 56

exercise 9, 43, 55

Fact Box 24, 28, 30, 31, 59, 60

Flexis 10, 16, 34

Food Intolerance .... 28, 29, 34, 39, 51, 52, 68 fruit 10, 14, 23, 29, 33, 34, 37, 39, 47, 50, 57

Glycaemic Index..38, 68

glycogen 29, 31, 54, 55, 68

honey 23

hummus 38

hunger 15, 31, 53

Hypoglycaemia...................28, 29, 30, 34, 39, 51, 52, 53, 68

ice cream..46, 57, 62

insulin ..... iii, 7, 24, 29, 30, 31, 32, 33, 34, 41, 46, 47, 67, 69

insulin resistance 69

natural weight...45

nuts 37, 47

Planners 10, 18, 39

potatoes.............10, 13, 21, 23, 24, 25, 27, 46, 54, 56, 58, 67

Quorn...26, 36

statins...60

Syndrome X...69

Tofu 13, 17, 26, 36, 40

Vegetarian.....................................12, 13, 17, 26, 36, 40, 58

71147456R00046

Made in the USA
Middletown, DE
21 April 2018